How to Lose Belly Fat

Quick and Easy Tips to Burn Belly Fat and Tone Abs

By: Crystal Stevens

Introduction

I want to thank you and congratulate you for downloading the book, *"How To Lose Belly Fat: Quick and Easy Tips To Burn Belly Fat and Tone Abs"*.

This book contains proven steps and strategies on how to get rid of stubborn fats around the belly and develop flat, toned abs. It's not a magic trick, and I don't promise an overnight success. But with the the right commitment, discipline, and perseverance, I guarantee you that you will not only enhance your physical form, but improve your health and change your life, as well.

If you are tired of being insulted by the way you look and you want to regain your confidence, I suggest that you start making the change now. Belly fat is no laughing matter. More than a nuisance, it can actually harm your body and health in the long run. Don't want until you develop serious health conditions before you decide to take care of your body and improve your life.

The time is now.

So, congratulations for making the right decision in getting this book! I will share with you easy, everyday tips that you can follow in order to lose those stubborn belly fats. It may seem difficult to follow them at the beginning, but as soon as you establish a routine and form habits out of the strategies, it will become easier.

It's all a matter of mindset. Always think that the changes I suggest are for your physical, emotional, and social well–being. Every time you stumble or hit a wall or think that "I can't do this", just remember the reason why you started—to enhance your body, improve your health, and change your life.

You can do this! I'm with you all the way!

Thanks again for downloading this book. I hope you enjoy it!

Chapter 1: Why Do You Have Belly Fat?

Belly fats are unsightly and annoying.

I'm sure you agree with me on this. And I'm also pretty sure that you can't wait to know how you can get rid of them now!

We will go to that shortly, but first, let us understand why you have a belly fat. Did it magically appear around your waist to make your life miserable and reduce your confidence in yourself?

There can be several reasons why you have belly fat.

Perhaps you like eating without being conscious of what you're taking in your body. Or maybe you spend most of your day sitting and not doing any significant movement. Or maybe you've given birth a few years ago and your belly just didn't go back to its original pre–pregnancy form.

Whatever the reason is, you know it. It's your body and you're aware of how much care you give it, or lack thereof. One thing is sure. The fact that you are reading this book means you want to lose your belly fat once and for all, change your body for the better, and improve your overall health.

So, congratulations for taking the first step! It may be a long journey ahead, but the moment you decide to go for it, you're already one step closer to your goal.

And since you've already started on this quest, let me be honest with you. Excess belly fat, medically known as visceral fat, is unhealthy and can cause serious health problems in the long run.

Understanding the Risks of Visceral Fat

Visceral fat refers to the unwanted fat in your abdomen that surrounds vital organs in your body, including the stomach, liver, intestines, and pancreas. It can also build up around your arteries, which can be very dangerous.

So more than a nuisance or an unsightly appearance, belly fat can really be harmful.

The more excess belly fat you store, the greater your risk for serious medical conditions, including hypertension, metabolic syndrome, type 2 diabetes, cardiovascular disease, and certain types of cancer.

At the onset, this unwanted fat you store in your belly can increase your level of insulin resistance, even if you have no history of diabetes. It can also raise your blood pressure immediately. If not dealt with right away, excess visceral fat can lead to more serious and even life–threatening health conditions.

How Did You Develop Belly Fat, Anyway?

You got pretty scared about the risks of belly fat, didn't you? Perhaps you want to know right away how you can get rid of it and just start living a healthy life.

We'll get to there in a bit, but before we do, let's go back and understand first how you got your belly fat in the first place. Knowing the cause can significantly help you prepare your plan of attack and identify the right strategies to burn those unwanted abdominal fat once and for all.

Here are the top culprits that make you gain belly fat.

1. Poor Diet

Wrong choices of food can drastically cause excess belly fat.

These include sugary foods, sweetened beverages, foods high in trans fat, low–protein diets, and low–fiber meals. Not only can they cause you to gain weight, they can also slow down your body's metabolism and hinder your ability to burn fat naturally.

Cake, donuts, muffins, candies, ice cream, and even frozen yogurts all fall under the high-sugar food category. Flavored drinks, juice, coffee, soda, and sweet tea are also among sugar-sweetened beverages that highly contribute to belly fat.

Foods high in trans fat, on the other hand, include biscuits, pies, cookies, margarine, microwave popcorn, frozen pizza, and deep fried foods. Trans fats are unhealthy fats. They are usually added to food in order to enhance its taste, improve its texture, and make it last longer.

As protein and fiber are important dietary nutrition that prevents weight gain, eating low–protein and low–fiber diets over a long period of time may cause you to develop excess belly fat and make it difficult for you to burn them off.

Are you a fan of the foods mentioned above? Are they part of your daily meals? If you eat them too often, don't be surprised if you're gaining and growing belly fat!

2. Excessive Alcohol Intake

Drinking too much alcohol may lead to many health problems, such as inflammation and liver disease.

In an article published by the Current Obesity Reports in 2015 about alcohol consumption and obesity, too much alcohol intake can cause weight gain to men, especially around their belly area. Other studies have shown that some components of alcohol stop the fat burning ability of the individual and excess calories are then stored in the belly as fat.

If you are a regular alcohol drinker, you may want to think twice whether or not to keep your "beer belly".

3. Inactivity and Lack of Exercise

If you consume a lot of calories through your favorite foods and drinks and you don't move around enough to burn them, expect that these excess calories will turn into body fat. The more inactive your lifestyle is, the more difficult to get rid of your excess belly fat.

The increasing rates of obesity worldwide has been linked to how people are becoming less and less active on a day–to–day basis. Because of technology and modernization, everything is becoming more convenient and within reach; thus, making people sedentary, sluggish, and lazy.

In a survey conducted in the US from 1988 to 2010, a significant increase in inactivity was observed which led to an increase in weight gain and abdominal fat in both men and women, too.

Do you enjoy being a couch potato? Well, you won't enjoy the fats sitting on your belly.

4. Stress

Do you often find yourself in stressful situations? Do you reach for comfort food when you're depressed or burned out?

Stress is also to be blamed for a fat belly. When you are stressed or under a high–pressure environment, your body tends to release cortisol, a steroid hormone that assists in body control and helps deal with stress. Too much cortisol can badly affect your metabolism.

Additionally, many people reach for unhealthy food when they are under stress, giving them temporary comfort that translates to long–term belly problem.

5. Lack of Sleep

Are you getting enough sleep every night?

Studies show that lack of sleep, poor sleep quality, and other sleep disorders, like sleep apnea, can cause unnecessary weight gain—which includes developing belly fat.

A huge study involving 68,000 women as participants observed their sleeping behavior and monitored their weight changes for 16 years. Upon conclusion of the study, it was found out that women who only had 5 hours of sleep or less per night had 32% more chances of gaining an additional 15 kg (32 lbs) of body weight than those who had 7 or more hours of sleep every night.

6. Wrong Gut Bacteria

There are many different types of bacteria that live in our gut, particularly in and around the area of our colon. Known as gut flora or microbiome, the bacteria in our gut plays a vital role in keeping our gut healthy, strengthening our immune system, and preventing diseases.

While some bacteria provide benefits to our health, others can disrupt our system and cause problems. An unhealthy balance of gut bacteria can lead to a number of health problems, including heart diseases, cancer, type 3 diabetes, as well as obesity and development of fats in the abdominal area.

In another medical publication entitled *Microbial Ecology: Human Gut Microbes Associated with Obesity*, researchers found out that "obese people tend to have greater numbers of *Firmicutes* bacteria than people of normal weight." This type of bacteria functions to absorb greater amount of calories from food, causing weight gain and development of belly fat.

7. Genetics

While we have control over the other factors we mentioned above that cause belly fat, unfortunately for this one, you may have to accept that genes and family history may be the cause of your excess fat around the belly.

We know that genes play a crucial role in weight gain and obesity of children. Similarly, according to a medical article entitled *Genetics and Epigenetics of Obesity* from the US National Library of Medicine National Institutes of Health, "the tendency to store fat in the abdomen is partly influenced by genetics."

So, if you don't want to be totally responsible about your current figure, you can partly blame your parents for your annoying belly fat.

8. Pregnancy and Menopause

Women have more reasons to develop belly fat because of conditions or health stages they go through, such as pregnancy and menopause.

Often called the post–baby belly or pregnancy belly, the saggy tummy of new moms housed a growing baby for 9 months, with an average weight of 7.5 lbs. And when the baby comes out, the mother's belly doesn't go back to its original form right away. It normally takes weeks, months, or even years for mothers to get back to their pre–pregnancy weight and figure—and that is if they're committed enough to get back into shape.

Menopause, on the other hand, causes belly fat due do a drop of estrogen, a women's hormone that signals the body to prepare for a potential pregnancy and start storing fats on the woman's hips and thighs. Without this hormone, the body will tend to store the fat in the woman's abdomen.

Now that you understand why and how you've developed that annoying fat around your belly, your next question would probably be, "How do I lose my belly fat? What are the exact steps I need to take in order to burn these stubborn fats?"

In the succeeding chapters, I will take you through three life–changing and health–improving steps on how to burn belly fat and tone your abs. These include:

✓ Improving your diet

✓ Doing the right physical exercises

✓ Changing your lifestyle.

Are you ready to change your life, improve your health, and lose that belly fat? Read on!

* * * * *

CHAPTER SUMMARY:

- Unhealthy belly fats, medically known as visceral fats, are the unwanted fats found in a person's abdomen. They surround vital organs in the body, including the stomach, liver, intestines, and pancreas.

- If not properly dealt with, belly fats can cause serious medical conditions, including hypertension, metabolic syndrome, type 2 diabetes, cardiovascular disease, and certain types of cancer.

- There are many reasons why a person develops stubborn belly fat. These include poor diet, excessive alcohol intake, inactivity, lack of sleep, stress, wrong gut bacteria, genetics, pregnancy, and menopause.

- The sooner your identify the cause of your belly fat, the sooner you can plan your attack and take action on how to improve your body and health.

Chapter 2: Improve Your Diet

The first step to losing belly fat is to reflect on your current diet. What have you been eating regularly? What constitutes majority of your diet?

You should be able to point out your nutritional problem areas by answering the following questions:

- Is it mostly made up of simple carbs from rice, bread, or pasta?
- Do you eat a lot of fast food?
- Do you constantly find yourself munching on salty chips or snacking on sweets?
- Do you always reach for a can of soda or a bottle of artificially flavored juice instead of water when you're thirsty?

If you answered yes to at least one of these questions, you may find yourself constantly struggling to get rid of your belly fat despite all the effort you put in the gym, strength training your abdominal muscles.

Nutrition and fitness experts agree that fat loss, especially around the midsection, is achieved through 80% dieting and 20% exercising. What you eat and the quantity of the food you ingest accounts for a large percentage of your success in getting that flat belly that you've always wanted.

What Foods Give You Belly Fat (Foods to Avoid)

Now that you know how crucial nutrition is in losing that belly fat, let's start by identifying the foods that you should avoid or limit in your regular diet.

Here are the food components that contribute to increased fat storage in the midsection:

1. Trans Fat

Trans fat is hydrogenated unsaturated fat that are often used to preserve packed items you see in the grocery. It prolongs the shelf life of processed food items, but it is very detrimental to your quest for a flat tummy.

Not only does consumption of trans fat makes you fatter than any other food with the same amount of calories, it is also believed that high amount of trans fat in your diet causes the redistribution of body fat towards the abdomen area, leading your body to store more fat in your belly than other parts of the body.

A calorie-controlled experiment on primates conducted by Dr. Lawrence Rudel, presented in front of the American Diabetes Association, showed results that diet containing 8% of trans fat has significantly increased body weight by 7.2%. Whereas the group fed with the same amount of calories, but with unsaturated fat instead of trans fat, had increased weight by 1.8% only. The difference is estimated to be much more pronounced among humans, which may put them at a higher risk in developing diabetes and heart disease because of its inflammatory effects.

Foods high in trans fat include baked goods like cookies, crackers, cakes; and ready-to-bake dough such as frozen pizza, biscuits and rolls. Some fast food are also known to use vegetable oil high in trans fat, so be wary of fried foods like french fries, doughnuts and fried chicken. Trans fat-rich margarine is also widely used in fast food dough like pies, pastries and other dessert items.

2. Sugar

Sugar has high calorie content with no nutritional value which makes you fatter the more you consume it—as compared to other food components with higher nutritional value per calorie.

A cup of white sugar is worth more than 700 calories, which means you may have to run more than seven miles just to burn that off.

I know what you're thinking— "But I don't consume that much sugar!"

Unfortunately, most products you buy in the grocery store are laden with refined sugar. If you are not careful, you may be consuming loads of sugar without even realizing it.

An average American eats about 19 teaspoons of sugar per day, that is about 2/5 of a cup or equivalent to 309 calories. A 16-ounce energy drink contains about 60 g of sugar, while a can of soda could have about 40 grams of sugar.

The World Health Organization recommends adults to restrict sugar consumption to only 25 grams per day. What's even worse is that most of the sugar you may be ingesting come from sugary beverages, which does not contribute to your feeling of satiety as much as solid foods. As a result, you tend to consume more calories unknowingly, resulting to increased weight gain.

Scientists pointed out that the high level of fructose in sugar and corn syrup is the reason why sugar should be avoided when trying to lose that belly fat. Fructose is linked to slower metabolism, decreased fat burning ability, obesity, and accumulation of visceral fat, according to a clinical study done by Stanhope and colleagues, published in the Journal of Clinical Investigation.

3. Refined Grain

Any dietitian, nutritionist, or fitness coach will tell you how counter–productive it is to eat refined carbs when trying to lose weight. It is also linked to several other physical and mental health concerns like obesity, allergies, weak immune system, exhaustion, depression, and anxiety.

Refined carbohydrates in wheat and white flour like those found in white bread, processed cereals, pasta, and rice have lost most nutritional values as a result of food processing. The food process that often involves bleaching of the grains strips away the natural protein, fiber, and other nutrition, making the resulting processed product harmful.

On the other hand, whole wheat and other grains, such as corn and rice, are not bad for your health and your goal to a flatter tummy.

Refined carbs will not make you feel full as much as the whole grain alternatives, which may drive you to compensate and consume more calories. Refined carbs have been reported to mess with your appetite and your blood sugar, making you crave more. A study published in the Journal of Nutrition reported that people who opt to eat the whole grain sources of carbs are less likely to have excess visceral fat compared to those who mostly eat refined carbs.

Furthermore, refined carbs have also been identified to contribute to other conditions that make your midsection appear bigger such as bloating, water retention, and constipation

What Foods Help Burn Belly Fat (Foods to Consume)

Now that you are all caught up on the foods that you need to avoid to lose that stubborn belly fat, let's move on to what you should be consuming to help you on your quest towards the perfect waistline.

1. **Water**

Water's role in facilitating weight loss and fat reduction is three fold.

First, drinking water throughout the day and prior to eating meals gives you the feeling of satiety. As a result, you tend to eat less food leading to fewer calorie consumption and fat burning. Drink a full glass of water before each meal to keep you from overeating during breakfast or dinner. Water has zero calories but gives you the feeling of being full, preventing you from snacking in between meals.

Second, drinking cold water has been posited to help burn more calories and to increase metabolic rate. Your body uses up more energy to warm up the cold water you drink; as a result, you burn more calories as compared to the calories you burn when drinking room temperature water.

Third, drinking water instead of soda or other sugary beverages will save you from consuming too much sugar and calories; hence, keeping you from consuming too much calories from your liquid intake. Fewer calories mean less energy to burn in your exercises or everyday tasks, which will signal your body to use up your stored energy, which are found in your abdominal fats.

In addition, according to a study by Murakami and others published in the European Journal of Nutrition in 2007, increased water intake is also helpful in reducing constipation among the people who have low dietary fiber intake. No constipation would lead to less bloating which will aid in making your tummy look flatter.

2. Soluble Fiber

If you want to flatten your tummy quickly, you may want to consider eating more oats, black beans, flaxseed, avocados, broccoli, sweet potatoes, lima beans, brussels sprouts, lentils, legumes, hazelnuts, guavas, apples, and blackberries. These are all very good sources of soluble fiber.

Incorporating more soluble fiber into your diet would help greatly in your mission to lose that annoying belly fat. According to experts in endocrinology and metabolism, Dr. Hairston and his colleagues, their observation of the consumption of soluble fiber in a span of 5 years revealed that soluble fiber intake is inversely proportional to amount of visceral fat in the midsection. These findings are published in the journal Obesity in 2012.

Soluble fiber contributes to the reduction of belly fat in several ways.

Firstly, just like water, soluble fiber helps you feel more satiated, which reduces your tendency to snack on high calorie foods. Soluble fiber and water work together to create the feeling of being full since fiber absorbs large quantities of water and expands in your stomach. As a result, you feel fuller longer for less calories. It also slows down the release of food from the stomach to the intestines, which means you will tend to lose your appetite because of your full stomach.

Furthermore, studies have pointed out that soluble fiber inhibits the production of the hormone signaling your brain that you are hungry. Fiber's ability to suppress your appetite will help in keeping you from eating more and snacking on high-calorie foods throughout the day.

Another way that soluble fiber aids in belly fat reduction is by decreasing the digestibility of fat and protein in your diet. In a study by Baer and colleagues published in the Journal of Nutrition, higher content of soluble fiber in the diet keeps you from digesting excessive fat, which means there is a lesser probability that the fat in your diet will be absorbed by your body and stored as visceral fat.

A similar study published in the Journal of Endocrinology and Metabolism showed that higher soluble fiber intake is linked to less visceral fat storage and lower rate of inflammation.

If these are not enough motivation for you to eat more beans and broccoli, soluble fiber also acts as the food of the good bacteria in your gut. As a result, it promotes healthier digestion. The process of how gut bacteria digests soluble fiber in the stomach produces fatty acids that have been linked to the reduction of fat storage in the belly and increase in fat burning.

As appealing as soluble fiber sounds for a person on a quest for flatter tummy, it is not recommended to abruptly increase your soluble fiber intake. Experts suggest slowly easing your stomach into the increased intake to avoid stomach cramps or diarrhea caused by a sudden spike in soluble fiber in the gut.

3. High Protein Foods

Digesting protein requires more calories than breaking down fats and carbs. Therefore, your body uses more energy just by incorporating more protein in your diet.

Considered as one of the most important nutrients for losing weight and belly fat, protein in your diet also increases the feeling of satiety, decreasing your tendency to eat more. According to Dr. Fallaize of the Nutrition and Metabolism Department of the University of Surrey, in a study published in the European Journal of Nutrition, eating a high-protein breakfast will suppress your appetite longer, keeping you feeling full the whole morning. Moreover, it also reduces the amount of calories you ingest during lunch.

Protein helps in building and retaining muscle mass and decreases the tendency of the body to store fat. It also boosts your metabolism and aids in fat loss.

It is recommended to have 20-30% of your caloric intake from protein. In order to achieve this, always incorporate a high-protein food source in every meal. A good source of protein is whole eggs. Despite the notoriety it received for having high cholesterol content, eggs have been proven to have minute impact on blood cholesterol levels. Eggs are packed with healthy fats and a high amount of protein, which makes you feel full longer.

Other sources of protein include salmon, tuna, almonds, milk, broccoli, Greek yogurt, spinach, lean beef, chicken breasts and other red meat, and seafood.

4. Coconut Oil

Although it may seem counter-productive to ingest more fat such as that in coconut oil to lose fat in your belly, the good kind of fat in coconut oil is viewed as very helpful in reducing the harmful visceral fat you want to get rid of.

Coconut oil contains medium chain fatty acids that are usually utilized by the liver as energy or ketones, allowing the body to achieve ketosis and burn stored fat. Studies have shown that fat from coconut oil are not stored in the midsection, unlike the fats from most foods.

Coconut oil is thermogenic as well, which means that the body uses up more energy to break it down, leading to more calories burned and increase in the body's metabolism.

Several studies have provided results showing how coconut oil help decrease abdominal fat and help control the appetite by providing a feeling of being full longer. This is because coconut oil takes longer to be digested.

However, just like any of the foods in this list, it is important not to exceed consumption more than the recommended amount. After all, coconut oil, just like other oils have calories from fat that may be counter-productive to weight loss when taken in excess.

Each gram of coconut oil has 9 calories and it is recommended to take no more than 30 grams per day or 2 tablespoons.

5. Fatty Fish or Fish Oil

Not all fats are created equal.

In fact, the fat in some fishes such as salmon, tuna, herring, anchovies, sardines, mackerel, trout, and other seafood like mussels and oysters have been touted as the healthy fat. These fishes are rich in Omega-3 fatty acids that are known to help reduce the build up of abdominal fat and help keep the liver healthy.

In addition, these fishes are also good sources of protein that helps aid in metabolism and in suppressing appetite as mentioned earlier. It is recommended to have two servings of fatty fish per week or take fish oil supplements to facilitate weight loss, and abdominal fat reduction.

6. Apple Cider Vinegar

Health enthusiasts swear by apple cider vinegar for its many uses and health benefits. One of these is weight loss and fat reduction.

The key component of apple cider vinegar that makes it beneficial is the acetic acid. It also contains other components like malic acid, citric acid, and lactic acid. Acetic acid in ACV helps lower the level of sugar in the blood and decrease insulin. Both factors aid in fat burning and weight loss. Fat and sugar produced by the liver has been seen to significantly decrease with acetic acid, thus improving metabolism.

Studies have also shown that acetic acid from apple cider vinegar reduces the rate of fat storage and also suppresses appetite by making you feel full, thus decreasing caloric intake. It produces the same effect as soluble fiber as it delays the emptying of the food in the stomach as reported by a study published in the Journal of Clinical Nutrition.

7. Probiotics

There are evidences that suggest that the composition of bacteria in the stomach may have an influence on a person's tendency to be overweight or obese.

In a study by Turnbaugh and colleagues published in the journal Nature in 2009, it was reported that a higher diversity of good bacteria in the gut are found among leaner individuals as compared to their obese counterparts. The strain and the quantity of beneficial probiotics may mean the difference between a flat tummy and a flabby belly.

It is recommended to regularly take probiotics that have been proven to aid in preventing and reducing the storage of fat in the abdominal area such as *Lactobacillus fermentum*, *Lactobacillus amylovorus*, and *Lactobacillus gasseri*.

Probiotics can be found in some yogurts, kimchi, and pickles, but there are many probiotic supplements that contain one or more of the strains mentioned above.

8. Green Tea

The popularity of green tea as associated with weight loss and belly fat reduction is not without merit despite the claims that the fat losses from regularly drinking green tea are negligible.

You should understand that drinking green tea *per se* would only help you in achieving the body that you want, but you should be mindful of the other foods that you eat and your level of activity.

Green tea on its own may have little impact on weight loss, but it facilitates the reduction of abdominal fat by supporting the body's fat burning ability when exercising. It also improves your performance in the gym by increasing your energy with very little calorie content.

Eating all these food and avoiding the ones that cause you to gain weight can only do so much if you have a sedentary lifestyle. Now that your diet is optimal for belly fat loss, let's look at the activities and exercises that will help you complete your quest for a flat tummy on the next chapter.

✶ ✶ ✶ ✶ ✶

CHAPTER SUMMARY:

- Food plays a crucial role in gaining or burning belly fat. This means you have to choose the right type of food items, dishes, and meals that you should consume in order to achieve a flatter abdomen.

- Foods that give you belly fat include foods high in trans fat, sugary foods and beverages, and refined grains. Avoid these foods at all cost in order to lose belly fat.

- Foods that help you burn fat include water, foods high in soluble fiber, protein-rich foods, coconut oil, fatty fish, apple cider vinegar, probiotics, and green tea. Include these on your diet and be on your way to a flatter tummy.

Chapter 3: Do the Right Physical Exercises

If you are eating all the right foods with the right quantity and avoiding all the foods that make you gain abdominal fat, then you are on the right track towards achieving that flat tummy you're dreaming of.

The next part of the process is for you to move that body more to burn calories, strengthen your core, and tone your abdominal muscles to reveal those sculpted abs.

Here are some of the exercises you can do to burn those stubborn belly fats.

1. Cardio Exercises

Cardiovascular exercises or cardio are physical activities that make your heart rate go faster and your breathing go deeper by repeatedly moving the muscles of your body such as legs, hips and arms.

Cardio or aerobic exercises pushes your heart to work harder to pump oxygen to your extremities, muscles, and lungs, improving your blood circulation. During this process you burn more calories and fat.

Brisk walking, running and swimming count as cardio. Competitive sports that make you move such as tennis and basketball are also good examples of cardio exercises.

To get the fat burning results that you want out of your cardio, your exercise should be between moderate to high intensity, and it should be done regularly. It is recommended to divide 150 minutes of moderate to high intensity cardio exercises throughout the week.

Cardio is important to burn calories and calories from fat, but it does not target your stomach. Thus, it may result to weight loss, but not necessarily from the abdominal fat.

It is important to target the abdominal muscles through strength training in order to tone the abs and aid in belly fat reduction. The following exercises do not need any equipment and can easily be done at home, and they all target belly fat by engaging the core muscles.

2. Planks and Side Planks

The plank engages the upper and lower abdominal muscles and helps improve posture by strengthening the back muscles.

To do the plank, get on the floor in a push-up position. Lower your upper body by bending your elbows to the ground. Your forearms and your toes should be supporting your body weight. Suck in your belly button to your spine and hold the position as long as you can. Repeat the pose for five to six times.

Side plank is an alternative to plank that targets the obliques, straightens the spine, and engages the core.

To do this, lie sideways with your body straight, hips and feet touching the ground. Place your elbow or your hand under your shoulder and try to lift your hips, thighs, and knees off the floor. Extend your other hand upwards to stretch your back muscles and make sure your abdominal muscles are contracted. Hold the pose for a few seconds and then repeat the same on the other side.

3. Sit Ups and Crunches

Sit ups are an effective way to strengthen the core by contracting the upper and lower abdominal muscles.

To do this, lie on the floor facing the ceiling. You can either bend your knees or keep them straight depending on which is more comfortable for your back. Put your hands behind your head or cross them on top of your chest. Try to lift your upper body to sit up using your abdominal muscles, while taking a deep breath. Slowly lie back down on the floor while exhaling. Repeat it a few more times then rest when needed. Try to increase the number of repetition each time with one minute rests in between.

Crunches are also very efficient in reducing belly fat by targeting the upper abdominal muscles.

To do this, start with the same starting position described above. With your hands behind your head, try to lift your upper back off the floor using your core muscles. Make sure to practice inhaling as you go up and exhaling as you go back to the original position. Repeat for a few minutes and rest in between sets.

4. **Russian Twist**

The Russian twist targets the upper and lower abdominal muscles and the obliques, which aids in reducing the stubborn side belly fat.

To do the Russian twist, sit on the floor with your knees slightly bent. Slowly lift your feet off the ground while leaning your upper body back. Hold the position when you feel that your abdominal muscles are completely engaged. Extend your elbows to the side and hold your hands in front of your chest. Twist your torso from side to side while fully using your abdominal muscles. Repeat several times then rest, and do a few more sets.

As you progress, you can increase the intensity of the workout by carrying weights or increasing the repetitions.

Doing the exercises while also maintaining a healthy diet, will surely have you shedding those unwanted belly fat fast. The next step in the process is changing some of your behavior or lifestyle that may be keeping you from achieving your goal body.

Move on to the next chapter to find out which habits you should start doing to have a healthier body and improved overall well-being.

* * * * *

CHAPTER SUMMARY:

- Inactivity or lack of movement and exercises, as mentioned in the first chapter, is one of the culprits in causing you to develop belly fats. It is, therefore, important to keep your body moving and engage in the right physical exercises.

- Cardiovascular exercises, such as brisk walking, running, and swimming, can help you burn more calories and fat. However, they don't necessarily target the midsection of the body.

- Workouts that help you particularly burn belly fat include planks, side planks, sit ups, crunches, and Russian twist. They target the abdominal muscles through strength training and aid in toning the abs. They require no equipment and can be easily done at home.

Chapter 4: Change Your Lifestyle

You're on your way to achieving the flat tummy that you're aiming for!

You are making sure you're eating the right foods, staying away from the bad ones, doing your cardio and your abdominal strength training.

But in order to make sure that the weight and fat you lost will stay away completely, it is not enough to commit to changing your eating and exercise habits just until you lose the belly fat or reach your goal figure.

The commitment to a healthier body should be a lifestyle. Along with being mindful of what you eat and doing your exercises, practicing the following lifestyle changes and making them part of your habits will help you maintain your healthy body and mind.

1. Avoid Stress

Keep calm! Don't stress it!

Whatever it is you are going through: work stressors, body figure frustrations, or any minor inconveniences, try to maintain your composure and don't lose it! Anxiety triggers the release of the stress hormone cortisol that increases your appetite. As a result, you tend to eat more when you're stressed.

So, make sure that you find time to relax, hang out with your family and friends, do what you love, travel, shop, and meditate.

2. Get Sufficient Sleep

To add to the de-stressing tips above, getting enough sleep every night work wonders.

Several studies have shown that lack of sleep is linked to obesity, weight gain, and increased waist size. The effect of sleep deprivation on weight is especially worse for women. Sleeping less than five hours a night has been reported to increase the tendency of gaining weight. So, make sure that you are getting seven to eight hours of sleep night after night.

3. Do More Physical Activities

Whenever you find an opportunity to exercise your muscles in your everyday activities, do it. Not only will it burn more calories, but it will also increase the endurance of your muscles, improve your blood circulation, and prevent the accumulation of fat.

Try using the stairs instead of the elevator. Or use your bicycle going to work instead of driving.

Additionally, when doing your arm or back exercises in the gym, do it standing up instead of sitting down.

Furthermore, studies revealed that you need at least 30 minutes of walking each day to prevent the accumulation of body fat in the midsection. Any little physical activity everyday will help you in your goal to achieve that perfect waistline.

4. Don't Skip Meals

Most people skip meals thinking that it will significantly decrease their caloric intake. However, experts do not recommend skipping meals or drastic decrease in daily calories.

Doing so would be counterproductive to your goal since your body will sense the lack of nutrition as a form of environmental threat such as famine. The body responds to this threat by storing fat in order to use as energy in the future when there is shortage of food. As a result, you may be slowing down your own metabolism by restricting yourself of calories by skipping meals.

5. Try Intermittent Fasting

You can consider doing intermittent fasting, which, when done correctly will burn off the stored fat immediately.

This involves eating your meals in a 6-10 hour window everyday and fasting for the remaining hours of the day. The diet should work since you will be burning the stored fat towards the end of your fasting hours, when your body has fully consumed the energy from food you ate during your feeding window.

Before you do this, though, make sure your are equipped with the right knowledge and best practices. Consulting with your dietitian or doctor is still the best way to go.

6. Avoid Distracted Eating

Eating without distractions allows you to focus on your food and how you are feeling. It will give you the ability to gauge yourself when you are hungry or when you are full.

If you often eat while doing other activities like watching on your cellphone, working, or chatting, you often miss your biological cues when you are full, thus, leading you to overeat.

7. Stay Positive and Dedicated

Lastly, it is important to keep a positive attitude and be patient. You will most likely see results of your effort weeks or months from now, so don't lose hope. Maintain your commitment to a healthier body and a healthy mind. Discipline does not end when you reach your goal waistline. Make it a part of your daily life.

Mindset plays a vital role in everything your hope to achieve. Train your mind to be positive and believe that you can reach your goals despite the hurdles and obstacles you face. A positive mind will push you to perform positive actions and deliver positive results.

So, don't give up! You've started this journey strong. Make sure to finish it right!

$$* * * * *$$

CHAPTER SUMMARY:

- Eating right and doing proper exercises are not 100% complete without making improvements to your lifestyle. To achieve and maintain a flat belly or toned abs, it is important to form healthy physical and mental habits.

- Among the lifestyle changes you need to make are: avoid stress, get enough sleep, do more physical activities, don't skip meals, try intermittent fasting, avoid distracted eating, and stay positive.

- Mindset plays a crucial role in staying dedicated in this journey. Whenever you face hurdles or obstacles, or you think that you can no longer continue, think about why you started in the first place—to enhance your body, improve your health, and change your life for the better.

Conclusion

Thank you again for downloading this book!

I hope this book was able to help you plan out your strategies on how you're going to lose your belly fat and achieve a leaner, healthier body. Understand that it may not be easy at the beginning, but having enough knowledge on why your body develops fats and what you can do to get rid of them is actually one step closer to achieving your goal.

The next step is to actually do it. Start making a change. Remember, more than an attractive physical body, getting rid of belly fat is for added confidence, healthier life, and improved overall wellness.

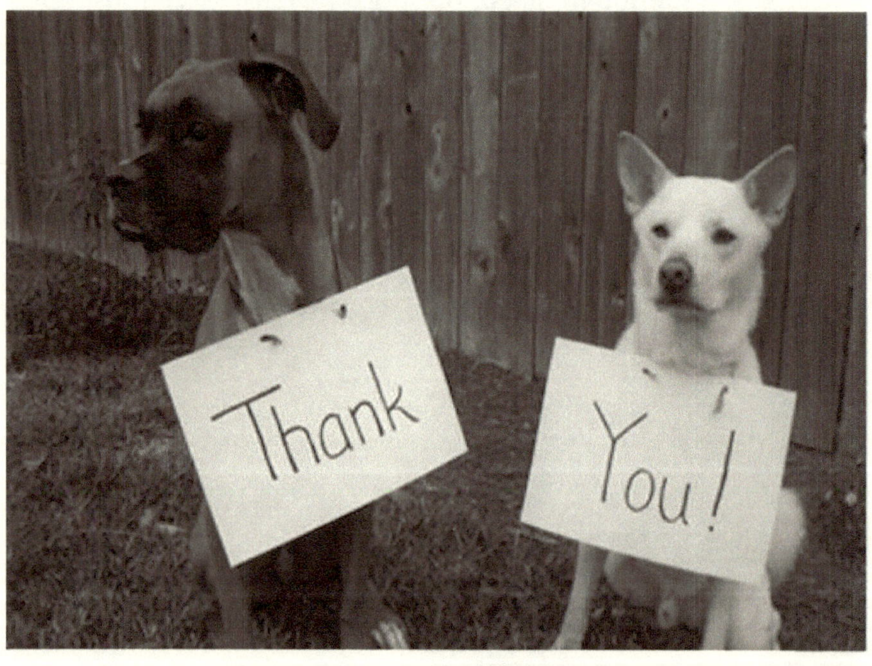

Finally, if you enjoyed this book, then I'd like to ask you for a favor, would you be kind enough to leave a review for this book on Amazon? It'd be greatly appreciated!

Thank you and good luck!